HEALTH HELPERS

SPEECH THERAPIST

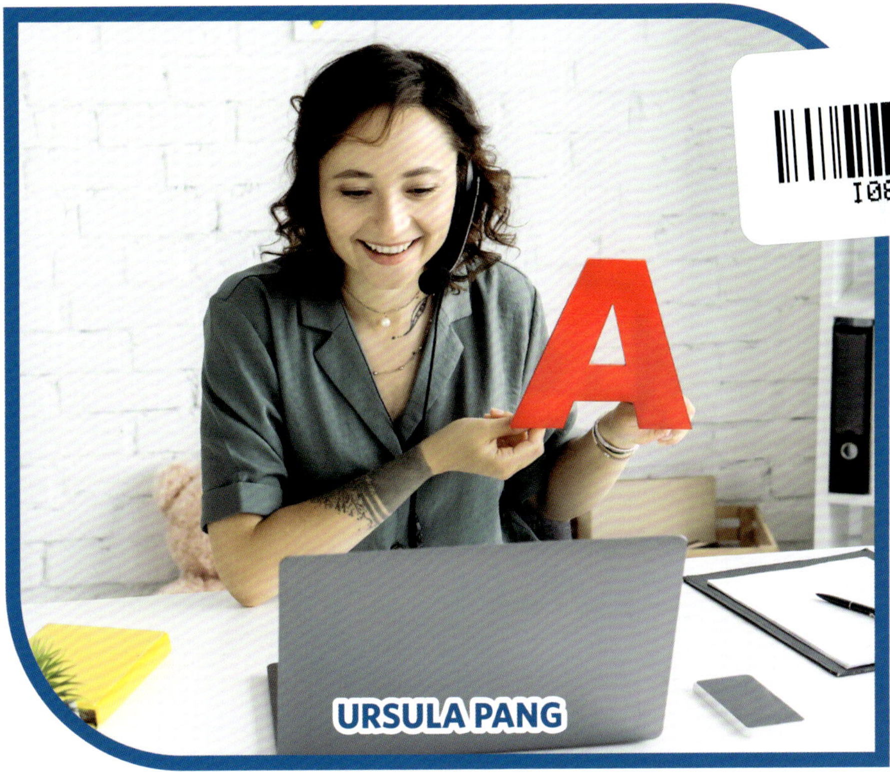

URSULA PANG

PowerKiDS press.

Published in 2026 by The Rosen Publishing Group, Inc.
2544 Clinton Street, Buffalo, NY 14224

First Edition

Editor: Greg Roza
Book Design: Rachel Rising

Photo Credits: Cover, p. 1 LightField Studios/Shutterstock.com; pp. 4, 6, 8, 10, 12, 14, 16, 18, 20 TechSolution/Shutterstock.com; pp. 5, 13, 19, 21 Pixel-Shot/Shutterstock.com; p. 7 fizkes/Shutterstock.com; p. 9 New Africa/Shutterstock.com; p. 11 Dragana Gordic/Shutterstock.com; p. 15 Miljan Zivkovic/Shutterstock.com; p. 17 Jelena Stanojkovic/Shutterstock.com.

Some of the images in this book illustrate individuals who are models. The depictions do not imply actual situations or events.

Names: Pang, Ursula.
Title: Speech therapist / Ursula Pang.
Description: Buffalo, New York : PowerKids Press, 2026. | Series: Health helpers | Includes glossary and index.
Identifiers: ISBN 9781499456554 (pbk.) | ISBN 9781499456561 (library bound) | ISBN 9781499456578 (ebook)
Subjects: LCSH: Speech disorders in children--Juvenile literature. | Speech therapy for children--Juvenile literature. | Articulation disorders in children--Juvenile literature.
Classification: LCC RJ496.S7 P36 2026 | DDC 618.92855-dc23

Manufactured in China

CPSIA Compliance Information: Batch #QWPK26. For Further Information contact Rosen Publishing at 1-800-237-9932.

CONTENTS

Let's Talk

A speech therapist is someone who helps people become better at talking and using **language** skills. These things can be hard for some. Often, people with speech problems just need a little help. Speech therapists are health care workers who help us **communicate** with ease!

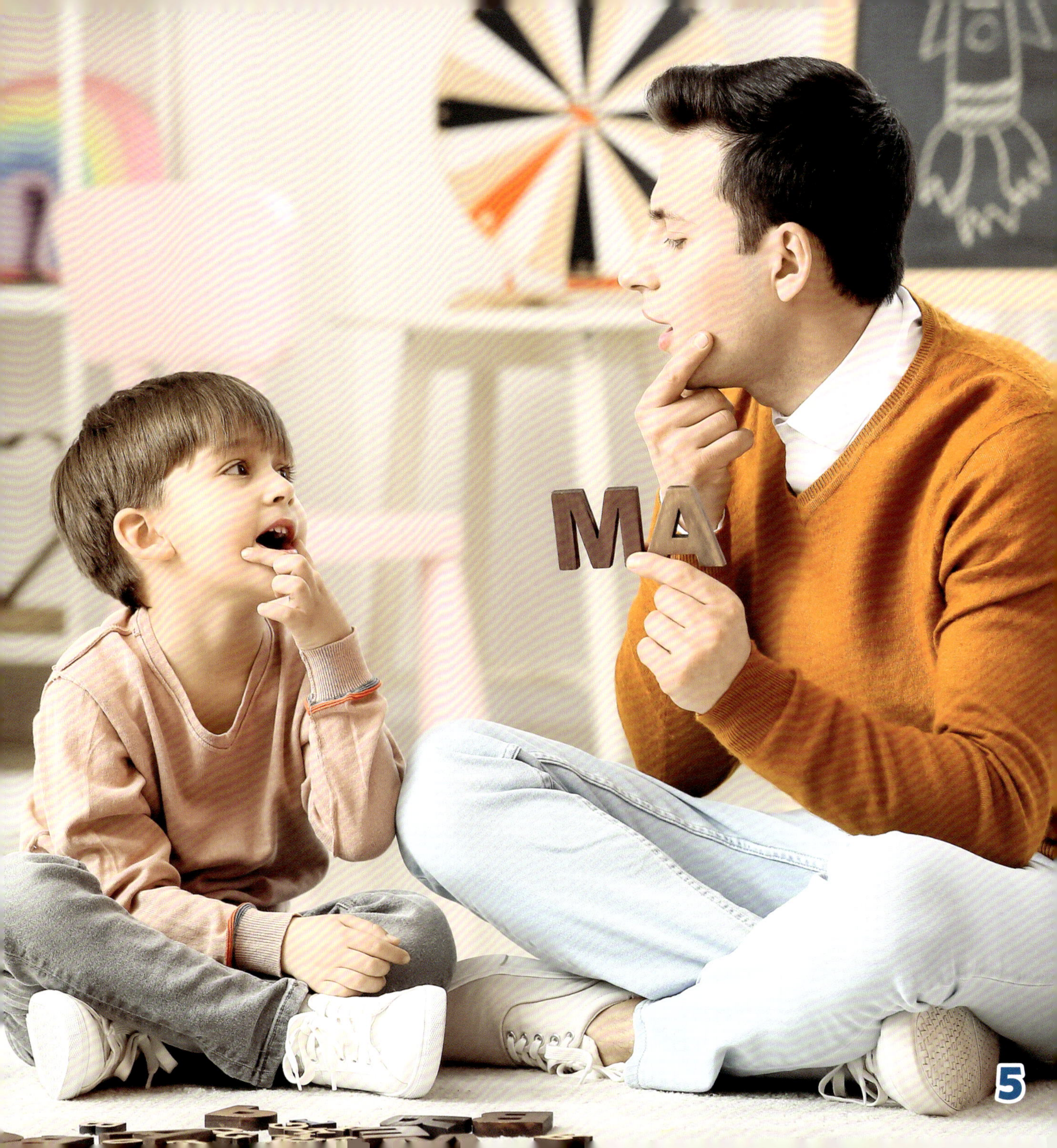
MA

Who Needs Speech Therapy?

A speech therapist will see several **patients** every day. They help people with hearing problems to form words they can't hear. They help people with birth **defects**, such as a **cleft lip**. They may also help people who have trouble breathing or swallowing, which can affect speech.

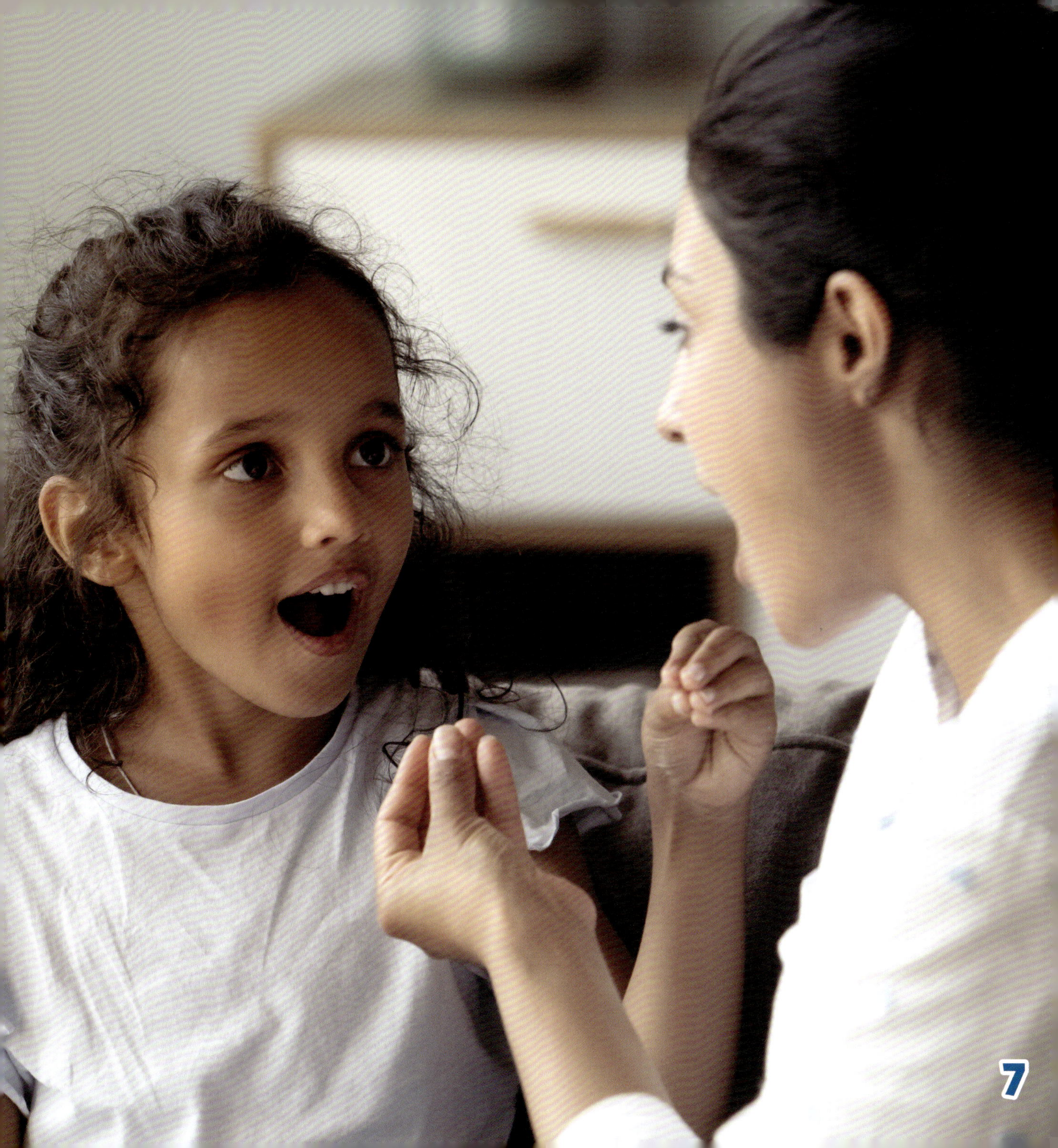

Getting to Know You

When you first go to a speech therapist, they will ask you questions. They will have you say some sounds and words. This will help the speech therapist find out what type of treatment will be best. This is a good time for you to ask questions too.

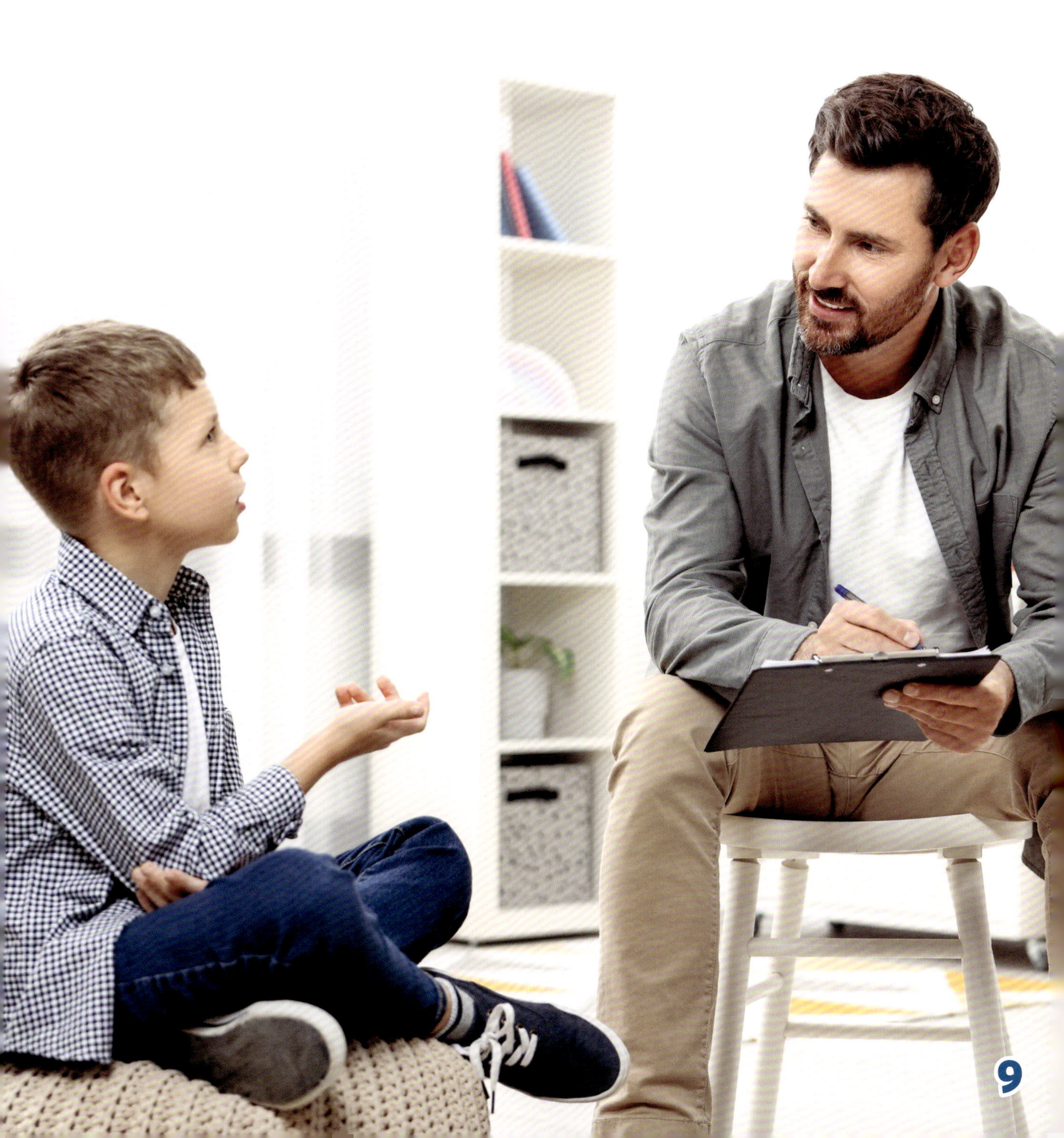

What Is Lisping?

Some people have trouble **pronouncing** words the way most people do. Some people have a lisp. That person might pronounce the word "sun" as "thun." Speech therapists help patients learn where their lips and tongue should be when pronouncing words.

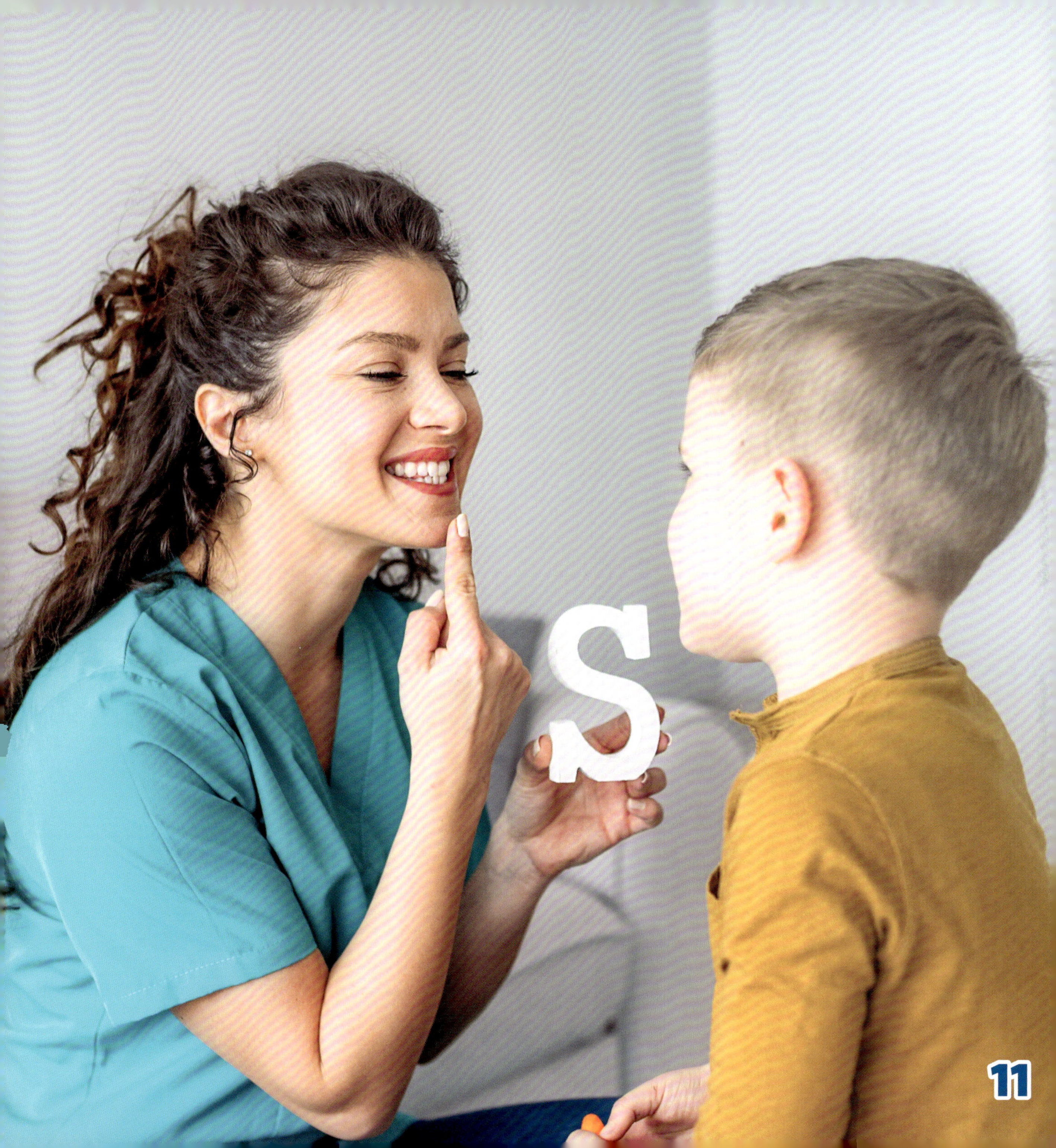

What Is Stuttering?

People with a stutter repeat sounds or words when speaking. When trying to say "sun," they might say "suh-suh-sun." The speech therapist may ask you to speak very slowly in front of a mirror so you hear each word and see how to form words with your mouth.

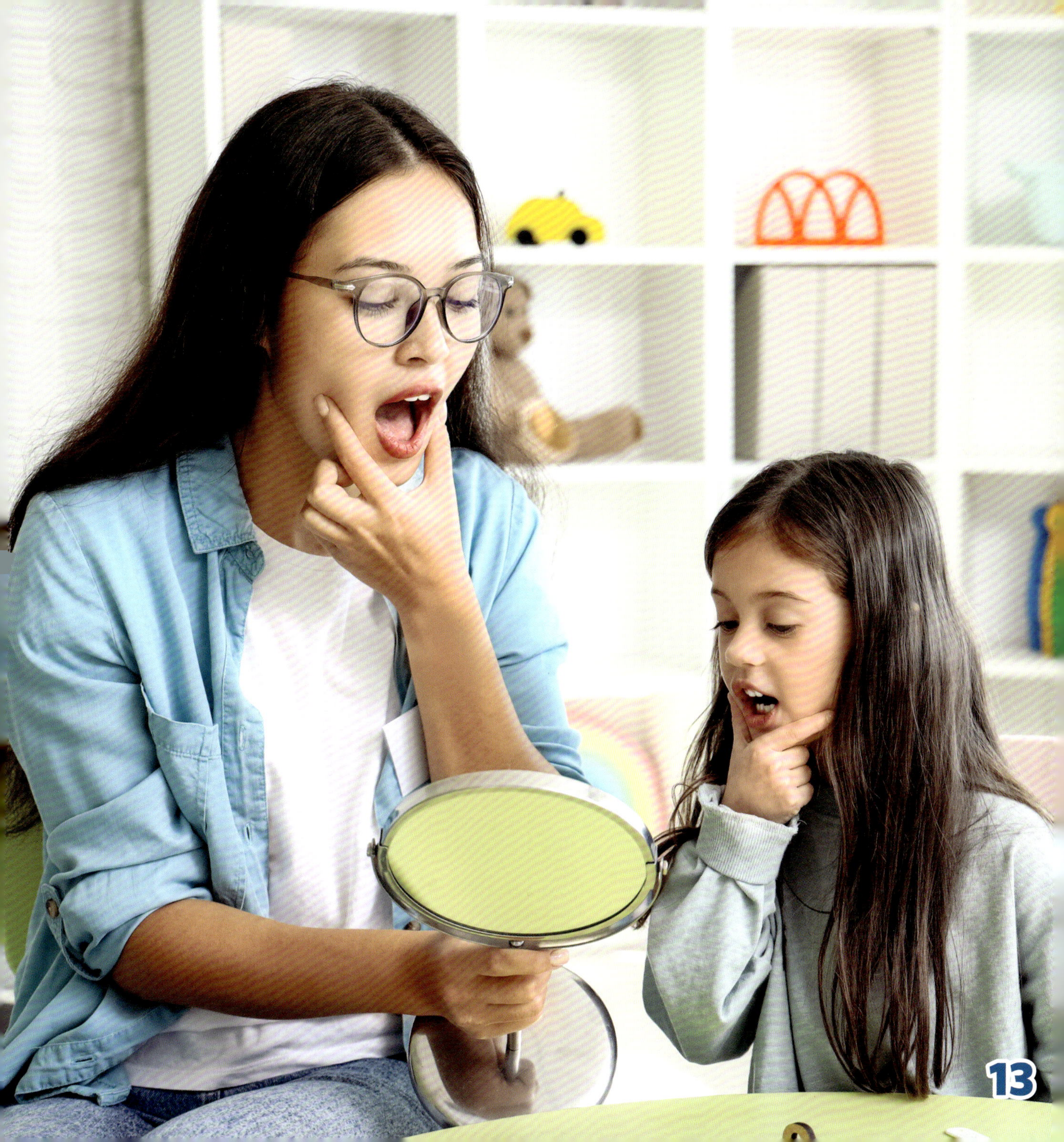

What Is Cluttering?

Cluttering means speaking in a way that is hard to understand. A person might say "uhm" a lot. They may talk quickly. They may repeat words, or put words in the wrong order. Treatment for cluttering is much the same as it is for stuttering and lisping.

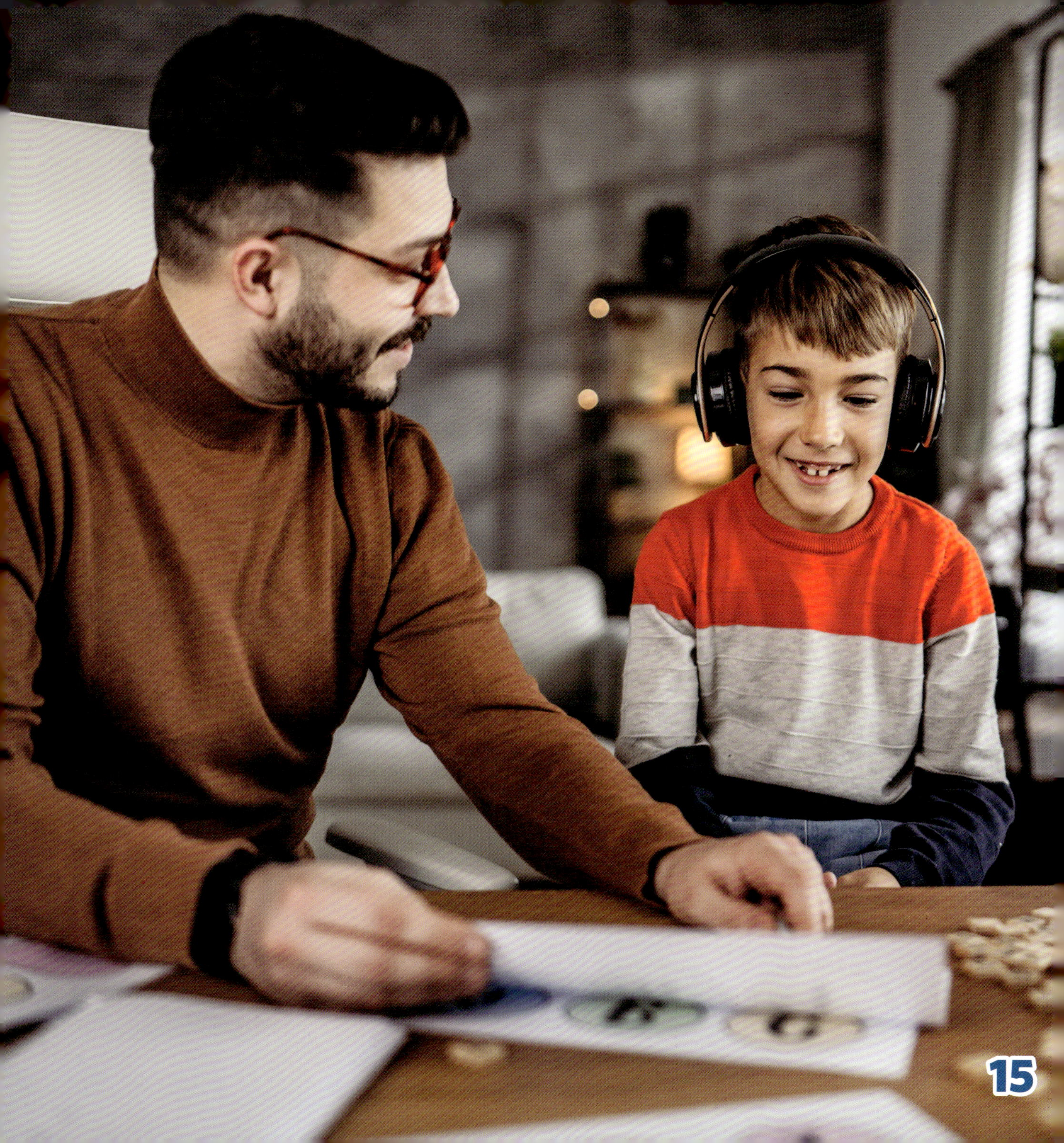

Tools of the Trade

Speech therapists may use tools to help their patients. Books, recordings, and toys are commonly used with children. A speech therapist may have you use an **app** to **practice** forming words correctly. You may even be able to meet with your speech therapist online.

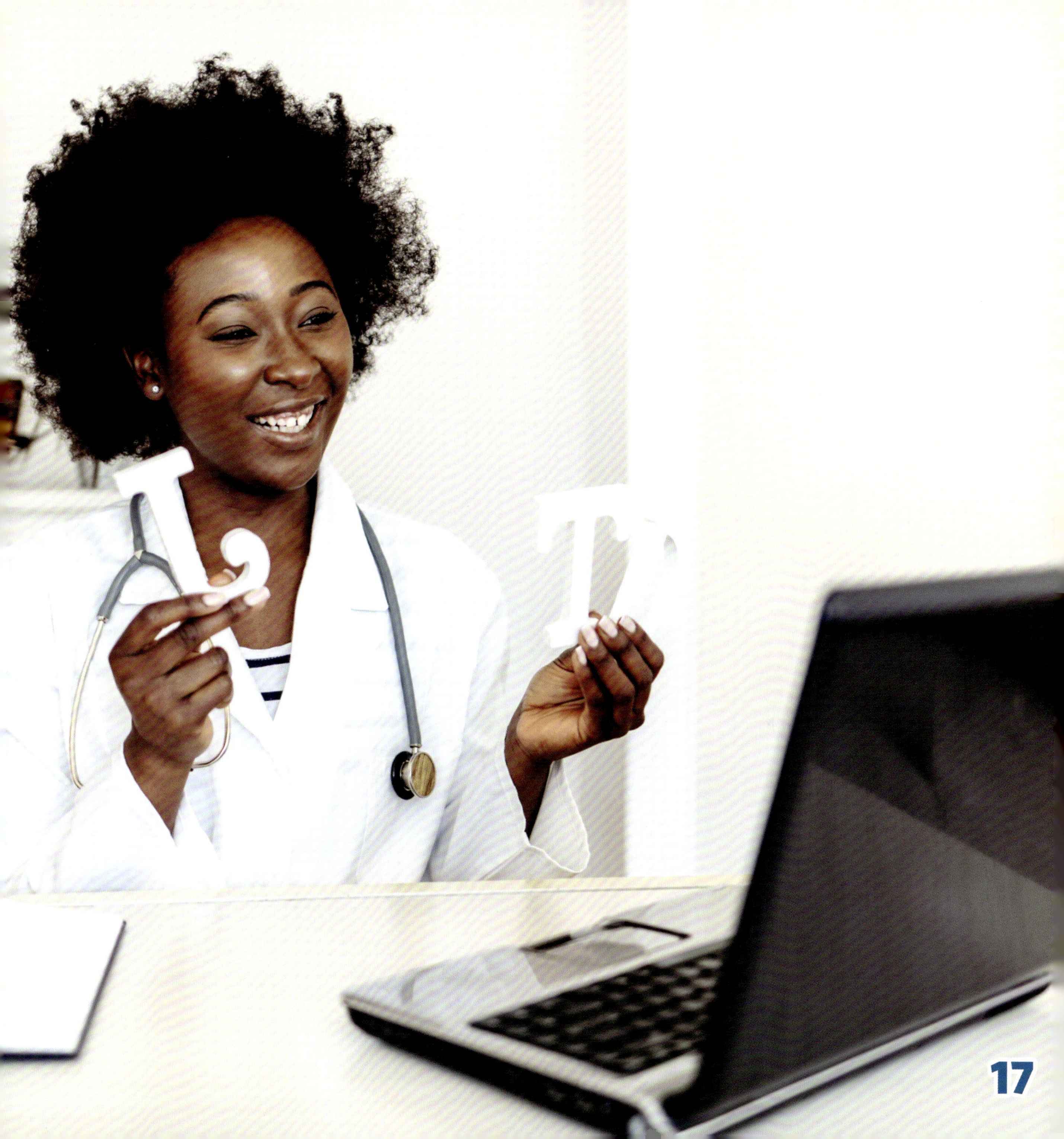

How Long?

The length of treatment can be a week, a few months, or a year. Sometimes even longer. Some patients see their therapist a few times a week. This could be in school or outside school. The speech therapist will help you practice and ask you to practice on your own.

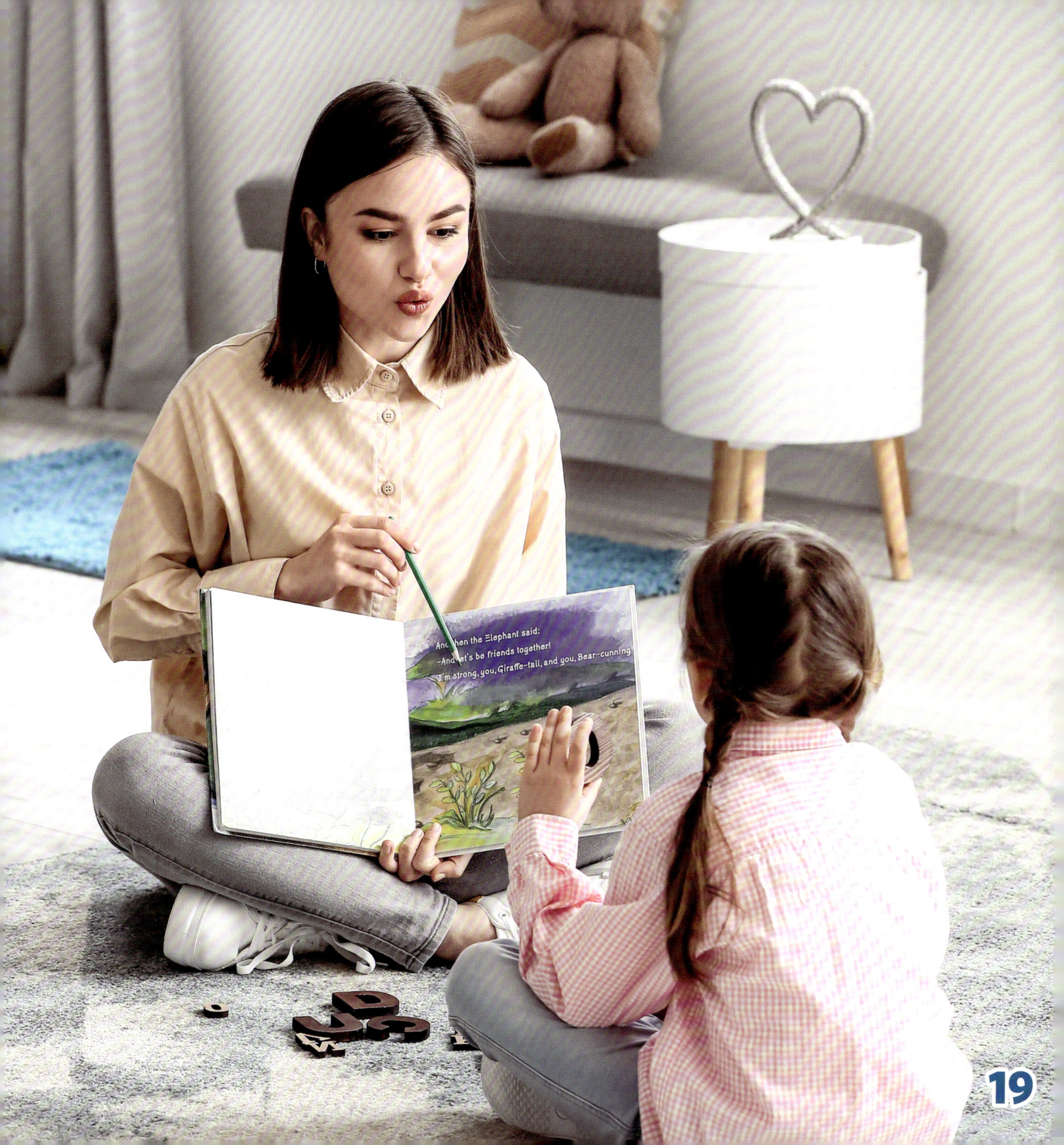
the Elephant said:
be friends together!
I'm strong, you, Giraffe-tall, and you, Bear-cunning!

Thanks, Health Helper!

Speech therapists are health helpers trained to help people communicate better. They work one-on-one with patients to make sure they get special care. They will even make their patients' meetings fun by playing games while practicing language skills. Speech therapists are here to help!

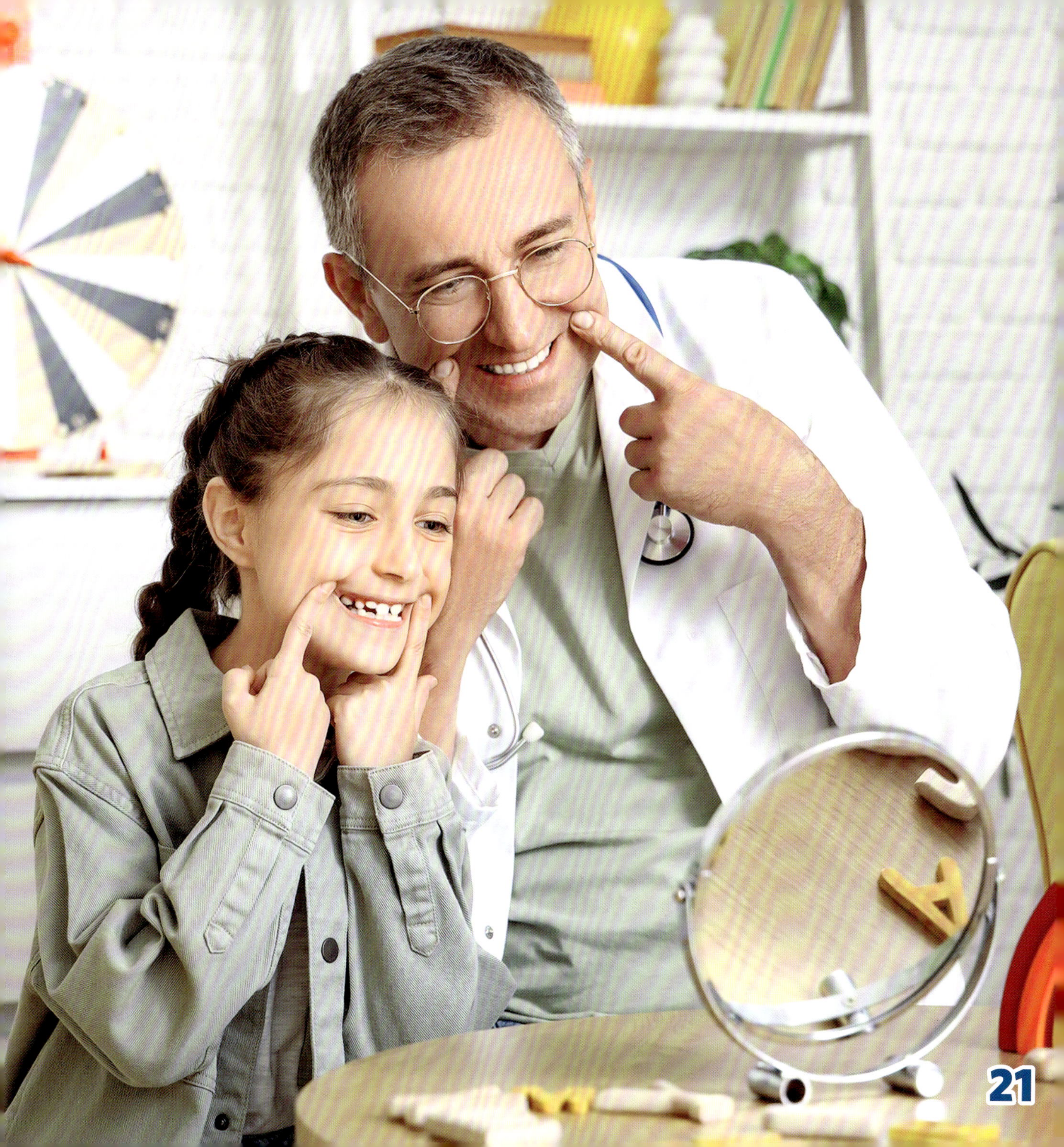

GLOSSARY

app: A program used on a phone or computer.

cleft lip: One or more splits in the upper lip that happen at birth.

communicate: The use of words, sounds, signs, or behaviors to convey ideas, thoughts, and feelings.

defect: A lack of something necessary for completeness.

language: The words, sounds, and ways of combining them used by a large group of people to communicate.

patient: A person under medical care.

practice: To do something over and over to become skilled at it.

pronounce: To say or speak words correctly.

FOR MORE INFORMATION

BOOKS

Harberger, Sandra. *Time for Speech*. Troy, PA: Harberger Speech Therapy, 2025.

Subrin, Liz. *Marvelous Margaux Goes to Speech Therapy*. Columbus, OH: Fishtail Publishing, 2024.

WEBSITES

Going to a Speech Therapist
kidshealth.org/en/kids/speech-therapist.html?ref=search
Kids Health has more information about speech therapists and how they can help.

Stuttering and Speech Problems
kidshealth.org/en/kids/stuttering.html?ref=search
This article discusses stuttering and living with speech problems.

INDEX